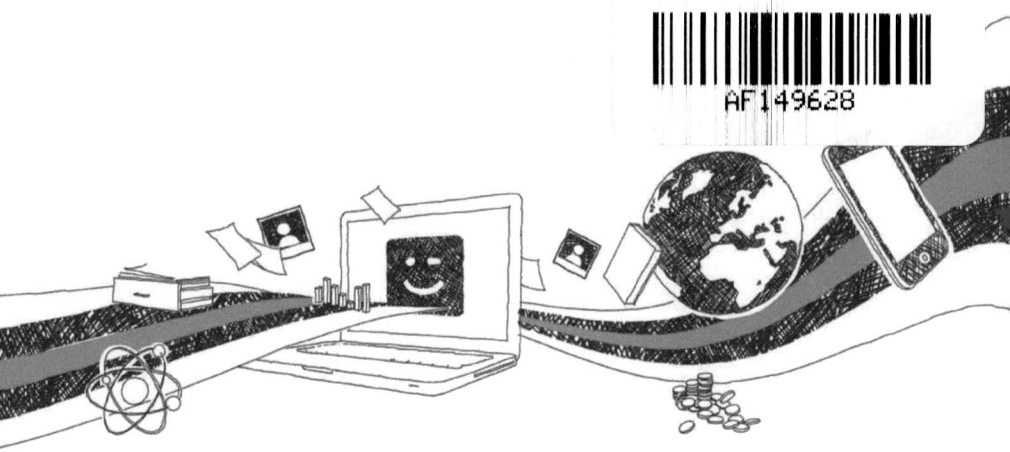
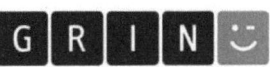

**Nora Demattio**

# "Memory Books" - Struggling against the Disappearance

## The Situation of women and children affected by HIV/AIDS in Uganda

GRIN Publishing

**Bibliographic information published by the German National Library:**

The German National Library lists this publication in the National Bibliography; detailed bibliographic data are available on the Internet at http://dnb.dnb.de .

**Imprint:**

Copyright © 2009 GRIN Verlag GmbH
Print and binding: Books on Demand GmbH, Norderstedt Germany
ISBN: 978-3-656-10847-4

**This book at GRIN:**

http://www.grin.com/en/e-book/187458/memory-books-struggling-against-the-disappearance

**GRIN - Your knowledge has value**

Since its foundation in 1998, GRIN has specialized in publishing academic texts by students, college teachers and other academics as e-book and printed book. The website www.grin.com is an ideal platform for presenting term papers, final papers, scientific essays, dissertations and specialist books.

**Visit us on the internet:**

http://www.grin.com/

http://www.facebook.com/grincom

http://www.twitter.com/grin_com

# "Memory Books" - Struggling against the Disappearance.
## The Situation of women and children affected by
## HIV/AIDS in Uganda

Universität Wien

2009

Name: Nora Demattio

# Table of Contents

*Nothing has a stronger influence psychologically on their environment and especially on their children than the unlived life of the parent.*

Carl Gustav Jung
Swiss psychologist (1875 - 1961)

# 1. Introduction

It was the 1ˢᵗ of december 2008 at 9 o´clock p.m. when I turned on my television and switched to ARTE, to watch a documentary I had read about. It was called "Memory Books – Damit du mich nie vergisst". I wanted to give it a try although I expected another depressing representation of "Africa" suffering from and dying of HIV/AIDS, as it has been almost common on the World AIDS Day.

It didn´t fulfill my expectations, in no way. I was touched, I was inspired and I wanted to know more about the situation of especially women and children affected by HIV/AIDS and the "Memory Project" of Uganda.

On the basis of this *experience*, in this paper I will have a closer look at Uganda, at the situation of parents, in particular of women living with HIV/AIDS on the one hand, and on the other hand at the situation of the children affected by the disease and who are left behind after the death of their parents.

First I will start with an overview of HIV/AIDS in Uganda.

Then I will provide an insight into the situation of women in Uganda in association with the epidemic, also concerning the law on domenstic and gender-based violence as on of the main reason for new and disproportionate infections of females, and the impact on children.

Furthermore I will introduce the "Memory Project" and its core, the "Memory Books", which was started in Uganda through the national NGO NACWOLA (National Community of Women Living with HIV/AIDS), and point out the importance for both of them, parents and children.

The aim of my paper will be to reflect the situation of women and children considering HIV/AIDS, and to provide an insight into NACWOLAs "Memory Project" and its "Memory Books". I want to overview the structure and to give a review on the goals of this program, as well as on its offered possibilities and maybe inherent difficulties.

## 2. Uganda

Since the 1990s Uganda is known for its success in fighting the HIV/AIDS epidemic. In this chapter I will first give a short overview about the history of responses to this challenge and present some numbers and statistics about the victims until today.

The second part of this chapter focuses on the position of women and children. I will discuss the women's status in the ugandan society, and the problem of domestic violence as well as its crucial impact on the health of the female population concerning HIV/AIDS. And I will give a short insight into the growing Orphans and Vulnerable Children (OVC) crises.

### 2.1 HIV/AIDS in Uganda

*"After escaping the bullets and the guns, AIDS was here. After hope, the monster."*

(Miria Matembe, Minister of Ethics and Integrity, Kampala, Jan. 13, 2003, in Human Rights Watch 2003)

In 1982 the first HIV/AIDS case was identified in Uganda. Wichcraft caracterized the initial responses of comunities admist lack of clear government statement to HIV/AIDS. But soon after, in 1986, due to a very fast reaction of policy makers, especially because of President Yoweri Museveni who spoke for a strong leadership in fighting the spread of te epidemic, the first AIDS Control Program was established. It focused on providing safe blood and the prevention of HIV infection in health care settings. In 1992, the Uganda AIDS Commission (UAC) was launched for coordinating the government response to HIV/AIDS. (Human Rights Watch 2003; Uganda AIDS Commission 2006)

In the 1990s the percentage of infected people decreased steadily from 18,3% with some centers of about 30% to an average of 6% in 2002, in regard to the favourable prevention policies. (Uganda AIDS Commission 2006)

Now the prevalence rate is rising again. Primarily women speak out against the popular ABC approach mostly due to their lack of power and possibility to discuss safer-sex, especially in their marriages. Women are looking for an alternative, for a change in the society because the risk groups have shifted. (Das 2007: 21)

Currently are about 30.884.000 people living in Uganda, aproximately 940.000 are infected with HIV. 480.000 of them are women (15+ yrs). (WHO Working Group 2008)

## 2.2 Uganda - Your Women and your Children

*"I'm tired of keeping trying to change consciousness. We need to change the law."*

(Deborah Kaddu-Serwadda, Women's Rights Activist, Kampala, Dec. 10, 2002, in Human Rights Watch 2003)

Ugandan women are disproportionately affected by HIV/AIDS, as well as married couples, who account for 60% of all new infections. One and maybe the most important reason is the existance of unequal power relations in their daily lives, the frequent dependency of women on men. The most dangerous outcome of this is domestic violence, from with the state is failing to protect them. (Human Rights Watch 2003, Wakabi 2008: 285)

Uganda is party to international human rights treaties and ratified the Convention on the Elimination of All Forms of Discrimination against Women (CEDAW) in 1985. (Amnesty International 2007) In the Ugandan Constitution, Article 33(6) provides that "laws, cultures, customs or traditions wich are against the dignity, welfare or interest of women or which undermine their status, are prohibited by the constitution". (Ugandan Constitution 1995) Nevertheless there are still customary laws and practices which conflict the Constitution, as on inheritance, land ownership, widow inheritance, polygyny, forced marriage, bride price and guardianship of children. (Amnesty International 2007: 9)

The Penal Code Act of 2007 deals in Chapter XIV – Offences Against Morality - with rape and other sexual an gender-based crimes, for which is also provided a definition.[1] What is not considered or explicitly defined as rape, is forced sex in marriage, one of the most dangerous because live threatening occurences and forms of domestic violence considering HIV/AIDS.

Due to the payment of "bride price" by a man to the family of a woman he wishes to marry, perceived as purchasing his wife's sexual favors and reproductive capacity, man mostly see themselves entitled to dictate the terms of sex and to use force to do so. Violence, or the threat of violence deprive especially married women of the opportunity to negotiate safer-sex with

---

[1] "CHAPTER XIV—OFFENCES AGAINST MORALITY.
**123. Definition of rape.**
Any person who has unlawful carnal knowledge of a woman or girl, without her consent, or with her consent, if the consent is obtained by force or by means of threats or intimidation of any kind or by fear of bodily harm, or by means of false representations as to the nature of the act, or in the case of a married woman, by personating her husband, commits the felony termed rape.
**124. Punishment for rape.**
A person convicted of rape is liable to suffer death." (Ugandan Penal Code Act 2007)

her husband. Besides that, abandonment from their home by doing so or by talking about HIV/AIDS often appears as more terrifying for the female majority because of their economical dependency. So they acquiesce to their husbands' demands for unprotected sex. (Human Rights Watch 2003; Leclerc-Madlala 2001: 36 Agostina 2000: 20)

Even when men know, that they are infected they often refuse to use condoms "... because he didn´t want us to leave us alive to remarry... " or they they don´t want to admit to the truth, to the disease. Sometimes it is just the bitterness of being infected what keeps them having unprotected sex. They forbid their wives to get to know their status through testing, or tell them that it has been herself who brought the disease if the status was positive. If so, she has to fear to be beaten to death or evicted from her martial home. (Human Rights Watch 2003; Wilson 2002: 30)

Most Ugandan women secretly get to know that their husbands are infected, they attend HIV/AIDS clinics in secret, they join support groups in secret and live with the assumption of also having infected the children in secret. It is fear that prevents women from accessing live saving information, from being tested and from receiving HIV/AIDS treatment and counselling which could also have saved the lives of their children. (Human Rights Watch 2003)


In 2007 the number of children (0-14yrs) living with HIV/AIDS has been about 130.000. The estimated number of current living orphans (0-17yrs) due to the epidemic at this time was 1.200.000. (WHO Working Group 2008)

These are two of the dramatically results of the disease concerning children, partly because of the reasons discussed above.

Mother-to-child transmission (MTCT) could be prevented for one, if there would be sufficient ART for pregnant women. Unfortunately just 34% of them received ART to avert MTCT in 2007. (WHO Working Group 2008)

Then again, if the government would be able to protect women from their violent environment by changing and enforcing the law in such a way that they didn´t have to fear battery or abandonment, and to equate their social status and rights to the of the male population, they would actually be capable to seek help, to attend a hospital for HIV testing and to hopefully receive the needed medication for prevention of, at least, the transmission. (Wilson 2002: 30)

Not only the number of infected women is rising, it is also the number of Orphans and Vulnerable Children (OVCs). Considering this, the Uganda AIDS Commission (2006) stated that "...communities perceive orphan care among the greates burdens of the epidemic."

7

Wilson (2002) already referes to this problem and points out that speaking of communities which will "cope" really means that women will (have to) do it. This will have consequences on the burden of reproductive work and in addition for the participation of women in politics, the economic sector, and so on. But the OVC crisis also leave children to take care of children which futher leads to less school attendence in order to work to feed themselves and their siblings. Girls will occasionally have to engage in survival sex.

The probably most devastating thing for children above all is probably the loss of their parents, their aunts and uncles, their family often without knowing what they were dying of.

Pamela Das (2007) dedicates an article to Beatrice Were, a woman who co-founded the National Community of Women Living with HIV/AIDS in Uganda (NACWOLA). She, like a lot of women do, discovered she was HIV positive several months after her husband died of AIDS. She had to fight with her in-laws to keep her property and her children, and not to be forced into marriage with her brother-in-law. When she went public with her HIV status in 1995 she reconized she had made a grave mistake, not because of her decision to do so, but because of not telling her children first. Here she detected the importance to speak with children about the diseas, to prepare children for bereavement and document their love, memories, to give advices and to post wishes for their future. Because of that Beatrice Were felt confident to start the "Memory Book Project", which until now remains successful and important, for parents as for their children.

# 3. NACWOLA and the "Memory Books"

In this chapter I will first introduce NACWOLA and its "Memory Project". Then I will have a closer look at the "Memory Books" itself.

I will reflect the importance of this work, for parents as for their children, and finally I try to outline the challenges surrounding it.

## 3.1 NACWOLA and the "Memory Project"

The National Community of Women Living with HIV/AIDS in Uganda (NACWOLA) was founded in 1992 in response to the desperate lack of information available to HIV positive women at the time. (NACWOLA 2009a)

NACWOLA promotes "positive living" through available- making of psycho-social support, economic empowerment and access to essential services including treatement. They seek to increase HIV/AIDS service uptake of HIV counseling and testing (HCT) and prevention of MTCT through involvement of women living with HIV/AIDS (WLHA). Furthermore NACWOLA challenges stigma discrimination and prejudice associated with HIV/AIDS and promote equal opportunities and speak up for social justice. (NACWOLA 2009b)

In 1997 NACWOLA started the "Memory Project" in order to support children who were facing the prospect of losing their HIV-positive parents. Its main elements are to train communication skills, to support in child development and parenting as well as in disclosing the HIV status, especially the children. Part of the project is also to assist in planning for the future and to give legal advice for women as for their children and in particular to stand by the children's side to help them dealing with the bereavement. (ActionAid Uganda 2009; NACWOLA 2009c)

The "Memory Project" aims not only to meet children's physical needs, rather to reach their emotional, social and spiritual ones. This indicates to strengthen their resilience through open communication between children and their parents/guardians, when they are able to express their emotions and fears, have a positive goal to live for. Furthermore supporting for their development is to give children the opportunity to help others, to get to a sense of resourcefulness and self-esteem, and to have them grown up in a supportive environment. The very importance to the emotional needs of children is also to have the chance to be aware of memories of the own past and loving relationships with the parents and those that care for them. (NACWOLA 2009c)

The "Memory Book" is an important part of the "Memory Project", and is seen as vitally important and therapeutic, not only for the children but also for their parents. For children it meets especially the last point mentioned above. The "Memory Books" have been created to strenghten their sense of identity instead of feeling deracinated, and help them to understand their family background and circumstances. (NACWOLA 2009c; Smith 2005)

### 3.1.1 The "Memory Books"

"Quite a few knowledgeable people adviced me not to bother taking the memory book to Uganda "because African people have an oral tradition and they won`t be interested in written words.'" (Carol Lindsay Smith, deviser of the "Memory Books" in the UK, London, 1990, in Smith 2005)

The first "Memory Book" was produced in 1991, as a response to the needs of African parents who had HIV/AIDS and were living in London, away from their extended families. These parents had been using the service of Bernardo`s "Positive Orphans", an HIV-specific project built to encourage parents to make plans for the future of their children. (Smith 2005)

In 1995 the "Memory Books"reached Uganda. One of Carol L. Smiths first contacts was Beatrice Were, who was at that time National Co-ordinator of NACWOLA. She, like most of the members lived openly with HIV, defying prejudice and physical threats but they all struggeled with the problem of disclosing to their own children, which inhibited them to plan their future care. Soon, with Batrice`s enthusiasm, the courage of NACWOLA members and the great support of the Ugandan government, the "Memory Project Training Programme" was started. (Smith 2005)

The basic idea of the original concept was that childhood memories are important in helping to determine identity and values as one grows older. (NACWOLA 2009c) Within communities affected by HIV, this is especially important. According to Beatrice Were "children can no longer learn their family backgrounds from their elder like it used to be in the past, especially because many HIV infected parents usually die when their children are very young". (AcitonAid Uganda 2009)

Using the "Memory Books", parents are able to tell the family history, can pass on traditions and values. They have the opportunity to express wishes and give advices for their children. For parents the writing process is also important to look back and to remember all the beautiful and happy moments they have had. The most books consist, besides the writings also of fotographs and drawings as well as of meaningful souvenirs pasted inside. (Graf 2007: 71ff; Smith 2005)

Being a significant part of the "Memory Project" the "Memory Books" can bee seen as a tool for communicating vitally knowledge between generations, and as a tool for testimony about HIV and AIDS. (NACWOLA 2009c)

### 3.1.2 The "Memory Books" – Difficulties and Possibilities

As writing is clearly one major part of the "Memory Books" it incorporates a problem for those people who are not easy on it. The adult literacy rate for females was in 2006 only 64.1% which indicates at first sight a visible barrier for some women, especially in rural areas. (WHO Working Group 2008)

For this reason some families have also developed "Memory Boxes" which contain objects of significance to the child and family. (NACWOLA 2009c) Nevertheless, the inability to write should not be seen only as an obstacle, many times it supports the aim to get togehter and to open up. As documented in Christa Grafs book and movie, in this case mothers will more likely sit togehter with their children, speak and explain while the children or other family members write these things down, ask questions and are able to add things the mother maybe wouldn´t have thought of. Also, as mentioned before, the book is not only for writing, you can find fotographs, drawings and meaningful souvenirs pasted inside. (Graf 2007: 173 and Graf 2008)

Were and Witter (2004: 141) made similar observations: "...Although the books were initially conceived as being filled in by mothers or parents, in practice children have been involved, especially where parents are not confidently literate..."

Although the "Memory Books" are encouragement to disclose, it still happens that parents die without speaking with their children, just leaving behind the book while many the mothers and fathers ask themselves "Why am I writing this down without discussing it with my children? Why don`t we do this together?"(Smith 2005)

Here I think Illiteracy is not a difficulty, in a way it can support to bring together the family, to open up much faster, and to involve the children in this process, in their lives.

Disclosure of HIV/AIDS is one of the most complex decisions parents have to make. Although there has been only little research on the effects of HIV disclosure on chlidren`s and adolecents`well being, the success of the "Memory Project" and especially the "Memory Books" speaks for itself. Children usually know somehow if something is wrong but they feel they cannot ask. (Bauman/Germann 2005: 104)

An argument for disclosure is also that not telling, secrecy, can have negative consequences for children. When parents do not tell them and explain the disease, they may imagine scenarios worse than the truth. Younger children may feel that the problem is their fault, or maybe they actually get to know about the HIV diagnosis and would need somebody to talk about. If parents or other adults have lied about the infection, denying that the parent has HIV/AIDS, the child will possibly feel betrayed and may grow to distrust all adults. (Bauman/Germann 2005: 105)

Of course, one may find some reasons against HIV disclosure but none of them justifies the harm that is done to a child, loosing their parents without knowing why, facing to grow up deracinated.

The disclosure also incorporates talking about death. While Bauman and Germann (2005) point out that it is reported that open discussion of death can be fulfilling and can increase cohesion among family members, they state also that it might be more difficult, amongst other, in sub-Saharan Africa, where talking about it is taboo for being feared to bring about the death. They refer to, in particular around such a delicate topic, a high cultural sensitivity.

I would not directly speak against this approach and advice but I think it is important to mention that this project nearly didn`t get to Uganda and more around the whole continent, if Carol L. Smith had been intimitated and convinced by some "knowledgeable" people, that "Africa" would not be interested because they have an oral tradition. Hasn´t it been Beatrice Were who acknowledged the importance and the potency of the "Memory Books"? These "Memory Books" and the whole "Memory Project" are now a huge success there, and one of the most effective approaches in fighting HIV/AIDS, its prevalence and its stigma, through making visible and readable that people infected with HIV are not just "worndown bodies with a terminal illness, but vivid individuals with a unique history, skills, achievements and aspirations for their children." (Smith 2005)

We should also not forget that although it was said talking about Sexualtity, in order to decrease the number of HIV-positive people, in Africa would be very difficult because it was taboo too, but as the history has showen it was possible, notably in Uganda as on of the most famous examples. (Graf 2007: 76; Human Rights Watch 2003)

Cultural sensitivity is very important but sometimes, I think, it is just a fine line between protecting and segregating someone or something. Talking about death is a very difficult topic, just as well here in Austria, but in some cases you have to and you will overcome your taboos, or your fears, and develop. Why shouldn't we admit this "Africa" too?

# 4. Conclusio

In my paper I provided an insight into the situation of parents, in particular of women facing HIV/AIDS, and of children affected by the disease in Uganda. I gave an overview of the life-threatening conditions under which women have to live sometimes and how it has an impact on the increasing OVC crises.

Furthermore, following Christa Grafs documentary "Memory Books", I showed the importance of the national NGO NACWOLA as well as its "Memory Project" and its core, the "Memory Books" to enable a healthier environment for women and children, to reach their needs and support them.

Finally I reflected some challenges surrounding the work with "Memory Books", as illiteracy, disclosure of HIV infection to children, and death as topics about which was said it were *taboo* to talk about.

The aim of my paper and for me was, on the one hand, to remind of the still existing gender inequaties and inqualities in Uganda, which is, through its often occurence as domestic violence and martial rape, nowadays especially life-threatening considering HIV/AIDS. It is obious that "...*keeping trying to change consciousness*"[2] isn't enough, the government should finally change the law, in order to be able to protect women appropriate.

On the other hand, using the example of NACWOLA and their "Memory Project", I wanted to show the flexibility, openness and socialagency of Ugandan people - who in my paper happened to be mostly women - in order to help the weakest, to support a possible living with HIV/AIDS, or although being affected by the diseas like many children are, who have to grow up orphaned, without parents. These children, who partly write "Memory Books" with their parents, and receive them from their parents when time has come and they pass away, they do not only get memories, they get support and hope for the future which they will maybe likewise pass on and re-stabilize a shattered generation.

---

[2] Deborah Kaddu-Serwadda, Women´s Rights Activist, Kampala, Dec. 10, 2002, in Human Rights Watch 2003

# References

ActionAid Uganda
2009                    Memory Book Projekt.
http://www.actionaid.org/uganda/index.aspx?pageID=1761
(09.02.2009, 21.40)

AGOSTINA, Ana
2000                    Carriers of Hope. / Portadoras de Esperanza. In: LOLA press, nov. 2000 – april 2001, No. 14: 18-21.

Amnesty International
2007                    Document – Uganda. Double Traumatized. The Lack of Access to Justice by Women Victims of Sexual and Gender-Based Violence in Northern Uganda.
http://www.amnesty.org/en/library/asset/AFR59/005/2007/en/60
68628b-a2bb-11dc-8d74-6f45f39984e5/afr590052007en.html
(09.02.2009, 17.30)

BAUMAN, Laurie J./GERMANN, Stefan
2005                    Psychological Impact of the HIV/AIDS Epidemic on Children and Youth. In: Foster, Goeff/Levine, Carol/Williamson, John: A Generation at Risk. The Global Impact of HIV/AIDS on Orphans and Vulnerable Children. Cambridge/New York/Melburne:93-133.

DAS, Pamela
2007                    Beatrice Were. Passionate Ugandan HIV/AIDS Activist. In: The Lancet, 2007, Vol. 370, July: 21.

GRAF, Christa
2007                    Damit du mich nie vergisst. Afrikas Kinder und die Memory Books. München.

GRAF, Christa (author and director)
2008                    Memory Books. Damit du mich nie vergisst. ARTE, 1.12.2008, 90 Min.

Human Rights Watch
2003                    Just Die Quietly.
http://www.hrw.org/en/reports/2003/08/12/just-die-quietly
(09.02.2009, 17.30)

LECLERC-MADLALA, Suzanne
2001                    AIDS in Africa. A pandemic of silence. / SIDA en Africa. Pandemia de silencio. In: LOLA press, may 2001 – oct. 2001, No. 15: 34-39.

15

NACWOLA
2009a                            Who Founded NACWOLA?
http://www.nacwola.or.ug/our_founders.html(09.02.2009,
21.40)

NACWOLA
2009b                            Living Positively.
http://www.nacwola.or.ug/+living.html (09.02.2009, 21.40)

NACWOLA
2009c                            Memory Work.
http://www.nacwola.or.ug/support.html (09.02.2009, 21.40)

SMITH, Carol Lindsay
2005                            The Origins (I):London, 1991. The Memory Book – And Its
Close Relations. In: Medicus Marcus Mundi Schweiz, 2005,
Vol. 97, June.
http://www.medicusmundi.ch/mms/services/bulletin/bulletin200
503/kap03/06smith.html (09.02.2009)

Ugandan Constitution
1995                            Constitution Of The Republic Of Uganda, 1995.
http://www.ugandaonlinelawlibrary.com/files/constitution/const
itution_1995.pdf (09.02.2009,18.30)

Ugandan Penal Code Act
2007                            The Penal Code Act.
http://www.ugandaonlinelawlibrary.com/files/free/The_Penal_
Code_Act.pdf (09.02.2009,18.30)

Uganda AIDS Commission
2006                            HIV/AIDS in Uganda.
http://www.aidsuganda.org/HIVug.htm (09.02.2009, 17.30)

WAKABI, Wairagala
2008                            New Strategies sought in Uganda as HIV infections rise. In: The
Lancet Infectous Diseases, 2008, Vol. 8, May: 285.

WERE, Beatrice/WITTER, Sophie
2004                            Breaking the Silence. Using Memory Books as a Counselling
and Succession-Planning Tool with AIDS-Affected Housholds
in Uganda. In: African Journal of AIDS Research, 2004, Vol. 3:
139-143.

WILSON, Shamillah
2002                            The Globalization of AIDS. The virus that follows
vulnerability. / La Globalización del SIDA. El virus que
persigue la vulnerabilidad. In: LOLA press, nov. 2002, No. 18:
28-31.

WHO Working Group
2008                    Epidemiological Fact Sheet on HIV and AIDS. Core Data on
                       Epidemiology and Response. UGANDA.
                       http://www.who.int/globalatlas/predefinedReports/EFS2008/full
                       /EFS2008_UG.pdf (09.02.2009, 17.30)